How to Burn Fat and Lose Weight Ridiculously Easy: Even During the Holidays!

Revised Fourth Edition

By

Gerry Marrs

ISBN-13: 978-1494425630

ISBN-10: 1494425637

See other works by Gerry Marrs:

How to Legally Rob Credit-Card Companies: Get Out of Debt Faster, Raise Your Credit Score, and Finally Live Free!

How to Write, Edit, and Self-Publish Your First eBook: Make Money Writing Instant International Bestsellers!

How to Make $800 Per Month: Starting Tonight! A "no-hype" realistic plan you can implement immediately, without spending a dime of your own!

How to Achieve Anything You Want: Set and Prioritize Goals, Attract Wealth, Live the Life You Always Dreamed

Table of Contents

Acknowledgements

I'd like to thank my two kids, Gary M. and Ashley who are a complete joy every day to be around and raise. Thanks for accompanying me on this life journey; I know it hasn't been easy.

Jeff Charron, whose talks on running and walking and the science of it all really started me on this path, and without your inspiration, this wouldn't be printed.

Introduction

Weight loss is never an easy proposition, especially if you are just starting a routine or even just thinking about the commitment it takes to lose weight. What many people fail to realize is that you can't beat science. The body operates as a perfect system of chemical processes and moving parts that must act together in order to create perfect harmony.

Sometimes, this perfect harmony is interrupted by things we don't want, like excess body fat, weight gain, stress, and feeling tired all the time. This is usually a signal that something is wrong with our body processes, and we must take action to get our bodies out of this condition or we face getting sick.

Similar to this though, interrupting a negative process is a good thing, such as introducing healthy routines into your life that will help you attain better harmonic balance.

I discovered that you can burn fat faster through walking, even more than running to your maximum heart rate. You don't even have to walk at a fast pace to benefit from this fat loss, your body chemistry does all the work for you.

In these chapters, we're going to show how different levels of exercise can benefit you in ways you might not have previously known, all by using your heart as a guide for exercise.

Many are unaware of the effects of stress on gaining weight and its harmful effects on the body. There are some things you can do to reduce these stress levels and this should be accomplished even before starting a routine. This book will show you how to do this through some very simple but effective methods.

Exercise is always perceived as a strenuous heart-racing activity; however, if your goal is to burn fat, you don't have to kill yourself and risk losing interest in a favorite activity. I hope this book gives you some great ideas for starting a simple routine that you feel happy about accomplishing every day. Just a little activity each day goes a long way.

One of the most important components of the ideas presented in this book involves tracking your heart-rate and your target zones. It's important to find a heart-rate monitor that fits your lifestyle but also provides you the feedback you'll need to implement your walking program. This book will provide a few ideas about what inexpensive types are available and some recommendations.

I hope you enjoy this book and successfully implement a solid walking program. This program doesn't have to be strenuous and can even be enjoying during a holiday like Thanksgiving,

15

Christmas, and other holidays where eating seems to take over the day! Living healthy doesn't mean living without, so enjoy life, live to the fullest, and enjoy walking!

If you like this book, please leave a review on Amazon to share with others. Thanks!

Gerry Marrs

Chapter 1 – Burning Fat, Not Muscle!

One would think that burning fat and building muscle take similar methods to successfully losing weight; however, surprisingly this is not the case.

Burning fat involves exercises that focus primarily on stamina and repetition, while building muscle involves the implementation of exercises that are high intensity and usually short duration.

Typically if someone is new or just starting out on a new program it is best to begin with exercises that focus on burning fat. This is because the biochemistry of our bodies operates in such a way that even if your end goal is to build muscle, you must first lose fat to start the weight loss process. If you are interested in burning fat, losing weight, and building muscle, then refer below to the aspects of those goals and how they can be achieved.

Weight Loss as a Gauge

Beginning with the end goal of weight loss is a good place for anyone entering into an exercise routine, which I'm guessing is the primary reason you purchased this book.

Psychologically, we get motivated based on the feedback we receive from not only others who you hope comment on your new look, but your own body as well, such as when you step on the scale and actually see your new program working. Current research suggests that even more important than losing pounds is losing inches around your mid-section (measuring around the belly for men and usually hips for women). This measurement is used as a gauge by many wellness professionals to demonstrate your relative risk for future health issues.

Warming Up to Your New Routine

If you haven't started a program yet or perhaps just in the extreme beginning stages you will need to increase flexibility before you go much further.

19

Your joints require ease of movement if you are planning to seriously implement weight loss regiment so let's take a look at some ways to start.

The best exercises to start with when beginning or resuming after a long hiatus are those that focus on strengthening the cardiovascular system but in a very light manner at first. These exercises include walking, jogging, stair climbing, and other variations of repetitious moment performed over an extended time.

You do not need to go to the extreme in this case.

The goal here is to build flexibility and keep your joints moving to the extent of preparing yourself for greater intensity in the near future.

Pacing Yourself Lower

When performing these basic exercises you want to have the main goal of pushing yourself to perform for as long as possible at a low level of intensity that raises your heart rate only slightly above its resting pace. It is common for beginners to underestimate how long they truly can perform an exercise, so it is beneficial to understand that there is a cognitive factor at play. Listening to music while performing a stamina based exercise often leads to an increase in both the duration of the exercise and the intensity level performed, due to the fact that it plays off of the aforementioned cognitive factor.

Music that motivates you may make you want to work harder; however, keep in mind that you may need to start at a low intensity to make yourself exercise longer, not faster and more difficult.

This leads to quitting early.

After you have had some experience with this low intensity exercise and increase in joint flexibility, you may find that doing the same kind of exercises every time creates boredom.

Variety = Muscle Confusion = Good

Establishing a variety of alternating exercises is important when mapping out a new routine. This enhances your performance by creating a new experience each time, and enhances muscle development by counteracting routine stress on the same muscle group. When creating this variety of exercises, you will want to assess your level of fitness development, as well as your desired end goal of burning fat or building muscle.

Focus on Burning Fat or Increasing Strength First?

The short answer is yes.

In the early stages, when you are focusing on burning fat, you may want to delay starting some exercises that focus on building muscle exclusively. These exercises include high intensity interval training; such as sprints and speed jump roping, as well as weight training and weight lifting.

While you can perform the aforementioned exercises and still burn fat, they must be performed in a proper manner that only someone with experience can accomplish.

Of course all exercise is good, the point is to start light.

Utilizing local resources such as gym and fitness centers and their services such as professional trainers are excellent facilitators to the progression of an exercise routine; however, in later chapters, we will show you a simplified, amazing way of burning fat with low impact.

More than Just Exercise

As you become more accustomed to the feel of exercising and watching your health actually improve, you may question whether there are other contributive factors that could lead to an enhancement of a weight loss and muscle building process.

Those questions are answered through the utilization of a proper diet and caloric intake program. Having a proper diet establishes a solid fuel system for your body and creates the setting for the desired goal of either fat loss, or muscle gain. In the beginning it is important to assure that you are taking in enough calories to fuel your body to perform your routine of established exercises.

Often, those looking to lose weight will simply decrease the amount of food they are taking in while not altering the type. This type of dieting leads to an overall detriment to your health and can cause many physical ailments. Assuring that you are eating foods that are high in protein, lean in fat, and provide enough (healthy) carbohydrates and nutrients to fuel your body are essential to developing overall better health.

Feeding the Fire

It is important to note that again as your goal changes from weight loss to muscle growth, so will your diet in both its composition and caloric amount. Typically when looking to gain muscle you need to take in a large amount of calories so that the building blocks are there from a biochemistry perspective to stimulate and feed muscle growth. Similar to hiring a personal trainer, hiring a dietitian to establish a diet plan that progresses along with your development is an excellent catalyst for growth and goal achievement.

Overall, if you are new to an exercise routine, it is typical to begin with the end goal of losing weight. This can be achieved through various exercise methods, but most specifically those that are cardiovascular in nature and focus on stamina and low intensity. As you progress and begin to lose weight you eventually will reach a point where you are in a target zone for muscle growth to begin.

Shifting Gears

This point is characterized by a decrease in overall body fat to a lower percentage and increase in overall mobility and physical stamina. Your diet should change to include more protein and some fat content, as well as increase in overall caloric intake amount. Your exercise routine should also change to now incorporate strength training through weight lifting and high intensity interval exercises.

As you continue to establish yourself in the exercise routine and become more accustomed to the variations of exercises you will find beneficial characteristics begin to appear. An improvement to your overall physical shape promotes well-being in the physical sense in your level of health, as well as in the cognitive sense with an improvement in overall mood.

Exercise promotes an increase in blood flow, decrease in potential physical ailments, and an increase in the productions and flow of the neurotransmitters responsible for happiness; dopamine and serotonin, which gives the end result of an overall better functioning human being.

The bottom line to this chapter is to begin increasing flexibility through repetitions and long endurance keeping the exercise light but where you can do more and for longer.

This is to prepare you to more efficiently burn fat when we implement the walking program described later.

In the next chapter, we will discuss a major contributing factor to weight gain that some people ignore until it's too late.

Chapter 2 – Lose Weight by Eliminating Stress

Research strongly demonstrates that chronic stress can significantly increase the chances of weight gain and obesity. When one is under stress, the body activates the production of hormones such as Cortisol (which affects the adrenal gland which helps the body metabolize sugar normally) and

Neuropeptide Y which causes abnormal growth of fat tissue.

Increased fat especially around the belly region is dangerous because it surrounds the organs, increases blood pressure and cholesterol levels.

How do you control stress-induced weight gain?

To prevent the risk of suffering from increased weight gain and reversing your workout gains when you are stressed, it is important to be cognizant of any bad eating habits you could fall back on as a crutch.

The following techniques can help you combat weight gain that is stress related:

Be aware of the warning signs of stress such as irritability, muscle tension and anxiety.

Do you feel flushed or do you notice your face in the mirror turning an unusual red color like a sunburn (this could be signs of a more serious medical condition)?

Recognizing the signs and symptoms of stress at an early stage and take measures to control them can be effective in reducing its effects.

Develop problem solving skills

Developing problem solving skills can help you anticipate challenges and simultaneously help you effectively cope with setbacks. Positive thinking about life issues is also another way that can reduce stress significantly

Practice relaxation skills

There are a variety of skills such as yoga, meditation and massage that you can perform to make yourself relaxed.

Regularly undertake exercises or physical activity

Undertaking exercises such as weight lifting, sit-ups, press ups and engaging in a walking program can significantly reduce weight for those already gaining weight induced by stress. Have an exercise program and plan on the time you are going to walk, run, jog or perform sit ups or workouts.

Find a distraction

When you are not hungry but feel like eating; you should find an alternate activity to keep you busy when you feel like eating without a reason, such as playing video games, watching an exciting movie or playing football.

Get encouragement from friends and relatives

Sharing and opening up to friends and family members on the things that are stressing you up can be a step towards managing stress levels. Family members can give you encouragement, support and advice that can significantly reduce the effects that might arise from chronic stress.

Getting adequate sleep

Having enough sleep is critical! Therefore ensure you sleep at the right time and for recommended hours. Ensure your sleeping patterns are right and that you have enough sleep at night to avoid stress caused by overstraining at work. Eight hours of uninterrupted sleep gives you enough rest which keeps your mind fresh and makes you remain productive throughout the day.

Stress Reducing Supplements

Persistent levels of stress can be debilitating and can sometimes be beyond the patient's control.

It is therefore advisable that when one reaches this level he/she uses some stress supplements available at various health stores.

St John's Wort for example is an alternative to the common antidepressants. It is mainly used to reduce depression levels in patients with uncontrollable stress.

GABA, is an effective supplement widely used now in controlling stress and helping one sleep. Some have compared it to an over-the-counter Xanax and have touted its positive effects in promoting peaceful sleep.

L-Tyrosine is an amino acid used to synthesize proteins but is now found to convert enzymes into dopamine. A number of studies have found tyrosine to be useful during conditions of stress, cold, fatigue, loss of a loved one such as in death or divorce, prolonged work and sleep deprivation, with reductions in stress hormone levels. This supplement can be found in nearly all popular health and nutrition stores now and remains relatively inexpensive.

Magnesium has been known to help relaxation when taken an hour before bedtime.

B-Complex (B6 and B12). During stressful situations the first vitamin to get depleted in the body is your B-series. Taking a combination of both vitamins will restore your energy and vitality.

Theanine is found in green and black tea, and may be used to relax the mind, tempering down the desire to feel angry.

Phosphatidyl Serine and Taurine are natural anxiolytics (anxiety decreasing drug) which work to increase dopamine and relax the central nervous system.

Following the above tips on managing and reliving weight induced stress is one step towards managing stress in both early stages right from its symptoms and chronic levels. A stress free life means significantly lowered pressure levels and long-term healthy living.

Next, we're going to explore how eating right can get you on a path to burning fat and losing weight.

Chapter 3 – Eating Right and Dieting

The key to gaining muscle and losing fat is eating correctly. The single most important element of every successful weight loss program is diet. You should pay strict attention about the foods you eat and the quantities. Your diet should be geared towards maximizing fat loss while at the same time minimizing any muscle loss that may occur as a result of the foods you take in.

There are four key points to remember when trying to lose weight through dieting and these are very essential if you are to see any positive results in your fat loss campaign.

A simple but proper diet involves

1. Eating foods low in bad carbohydrates
2. Closely monitoring your calorie intake
3. Ensuring you are receiving the proper vitamins and minerals your body needs

Limiting Carbohydrates

One of the most important ways to lose fat is by reducing intake of bad carbohydrates. The body

41

uses carbohydrates as the main source of energy. During digestion, sugars and starches are broken down into simple sugars and absorbed into the bloodstream. When they are absorbed into the bloodstream, they are known as glucose or blood sugar.

Some of this glucose is used by the body for energy while the rest is either stored in the liver, muscles and other cells or converted into fat.

The theory behind "low carb" diets is that insulin prevents the breakdown of fat in the body by allowing sugar to be used for energy. Limiting the amount of carbs you take in lowers insulin levels and causes the body to burn excess stored fat for energy. Ultimately, this helps you to shed off the excess fat. For effective weight loss, one has to stay under 20 grams of carbs per day. Avoid foods rich in carbs such as pasta, bread and rice especially when you have just started your weight loss campaign.

This is a very difficult lifestyle to maintain but does work for kick-starting your weight-loss campaign.

Counting calories the simple way

Another simple way of burning fat and losing weight is by counting calories. It is very important to take record of the amount of calories you eat and burn in a day. To be able to burn fat effectively, you must create a calorie deficit. This means that you must eat less calories than your body burns in a day. You can create a calorie deficit by eating fewer calories than you eat presently and exercising more or a combination of the two. This therefore means you must seriously monitor and track the amount of calories that you take in.

There are so many online tools available to help you track your intake.

My Fitness Pal (myfitnesspal.com) has an app you can download to your smart phone or tablet to begin tracking right away.

Key Ways to Track Calories

The tips below can help you to effectively monitor and track the amount of calories you eat or burn on a daily basis.

- Don't make it complicated. Use simple tools that are easy for you to understand.

- Use online tracking websites or download tracking software online. Such websites include www.fitwatch.com and you can download the FitWatch Fitness tracker to help you count and keep track of your calories on your PC or smart-phone.

- Carry around a small notebook where you record all the calories you eat while on the go. This can be helpful especially when eating away from home.

Why Fad Diets Are Bad

Fad diets have been promoted as a weight loss diet but on the contrary, they have been found to increase weight gain in some cases. They can be tempting but if you're trying to burn fat, you must try to avoid using them solely as a means of weight loss as much as possible. Here are some reasons why you should avoid fad diets;

- Weight gain. The main selling point of fad diets is their claim to help you lose weight in the shortest time possible and with very minimal effort. This sounds quite suspicious because weight loss is a gradual process. When you get on a fad diet, chances are that you may lose weight quickly because you will be on a restricted diet but the truth is that most of this is simply water weight. As soon as you stop the diet and begin eating normally, there are high chances that you will gain the weight back with additional pounds.

- Alters metabolism. Fad diets require you to eat a structured amount of food and this can disrupt your body's natural metabolism.

- Nutritional deficiencies. Fad diets restrict the types of food you eat and this deprives the body of some vital nutrients and minerals.

- Hair and muscle loss. The nutritional deficiencies caused by fad diets can lead to hair and muscle loss. Your hair requires plenty of protein for proper growth so when you're not getting enough of it, your hair will lose its health. Also since your body is low on calories, it will look for ways to get energy and one of them is by digesting your muscles thus leading to weight gain because muscles help to burn more calories.

Eating the right foods

For successful fat loss, it is also important to eat the right foods. You have to eat a proper mix of fat burning foods like vegetables, proteins, fats and gluten free foods. The following food types will be very helpful in your weight loss campaign;

- Vegetables. Leafy vegetables like lettuce, broccoli have very low amounts of carbohydrates and can be very good for those trying to trim off some fat. On the other hand, starchy vegetables that grow underground contain very high amounts of carbs and are not typically good for weight loss (potatoes are a known high carb food and bad for weight loss; however, they are a low-fat food).

- Proteins. For effective fat loss, you need to eat a lot of protein rich foods. Actually, proteins should take up close to 40% of your daily diet. Proteins help in muscle growth and repair. Foods rich in proteins include eggs, lean meat, whey protein and soy protein.

- Eat gluten free products. Gluten is a protein complex found in wheat, barley and rye. Striving to eat gluten-free foods and eating more lean protein, vegetables and fruits can lead to weight loss as it helps replace white flour, junk foods and sugar that contribute to weight gain.

A key word about vitamins and minerals; there is a minimum amount that your body needs to take in to operate normally.

There are 13 vitamins your body needs. They are

- Vitamin A
- B vitamins (thiamine, riboflavin, niacin, pantothenic acid, biotin, vitamin B-6, vitamin B-12 and folate)
- Vitamin C
- Vitamin D

- Vitamin E

- Vitamin K

You can usually get all your vitamins from the foods you eat. Your body can also produce vitamins D and K. If you are on a vegetarian diet, you may need to take a vitamin B12 supplement.

Each vitamin has specific jobs. If you have low levels of certain vitamins, you notice some negative health effects. If you don't take in enough vitamin C, you can become anemic. Some vitamins may help prevent medical problems. Vitamin A prevents night blindness.

The best way to get enough vitamins is to eat a balanced diet with a variety of foods. In some cases, you may need to take vitamin supplements.

It's a good idea to ask your health care provider first. High doses of some vitamins can cause problems.

Eating right and dieting is therefore very important if you are to effectively lose fat. However, you must balance all these foods in the right proportions. Starving yourself will do no good in helping you lose weight.

Anaerobic Methods

Weight loss is necessary for anyone who has excess weight. If you feel that your weight is not right, you have a responsibility to cut down the weight not just for you to look good but also to keep healthy. However, losing weight has to be done in a healthy way.

Other than checking your diet, you need to enhance the energy use by the body. You need to exercise for the energy to burn in the form of calories. This process is described by fancy names such as aerobic and anaerobic fat burning.

You may opt to lift weight, do push-ups, do sit ups or involve in other muscular activities. When you are doing this, you are involved in anaerobic exercises. Your other option is taking a jog, running on the treadmill, involve in sports such as soccer and other activities that keep your body breathing heavily. These are aerobic exercises. These exercises have different effects when it comes to getting your body into shape.

When exercising, calories are burned off from the fat and carbohydrate reserves. This results to weight loss as the accumulated fat is reduced by the burning effect. While the fat burns you get energy and you cut weight.

Aerobic simply means that the fat burning occurs with oxygen. In aerobic burning, oxygen is needed to facilitate the burning of fats in the body. The other form of fat burning is the anaerobic fat burning.

Anaerobic fat burning is the opposite of aerobic. It involves fat burning in the absence of oxygen. Oxygen is not needed for the calories to be burn.

Both aerobic and anaerobic exercises enable you to cut weight. However, the duration and intensity within which you cut weight varies with the exercise that you select. You get to burn the fats at different rates. You will select the appropriate approach to weight loss depending on your personal fitness goals. However, you have to consider the disadvantages of anaerobic fat burning.

Disadvantages of anaerobic exercises in relation to aerobic exercise

Anaerobic workouts are known to burn primarily glycogen. Anaerobic work out which involve weight lifting, push-ups, and sit-ups among other activities do not burn fats instead. This way, they are not as effective as aerobic workout when it comes to reducing the fat levels.

You will not reduce fat levels with anaerobic as you would have with aerobic exercise. It is slow and inefficient by itself. If you need to burn more fats within a shorter period of time, you need to consider aerobic exercises rather than anaerobic exercises. If you are exercising with the primary goal of reducing weight, then you should consider more of aerobic than anaerobic exercise.

If you need to make muscles, anaerobic exercises are for you. Anaerobic muscles are more effective in building muscles than burning fats. You can get to build more targeted muscles with this form of exercise than you will with aerobic exercise. On the flip side, you will be less efficient in cutting down on the body weight compared to when you are doing anaerobic exercises. You have to decide on your fitness goals and adopt the form of exercise that fits your intentions.

Anaerobic exercises tend to burn more calories from carbohydrates than from fats. While weight gain is usually as a result of accumulated fats, this makes it an inefficient approach to cutting weight. For one to cut down on weight, you need to get the calories from the fat deposits. You can trim your body and reduce the accumulated fats by burning the fats in the body. However, anaerobic exercises will convert the carbohydrates and the not the fat into calories.

When it comes to fat burning zones, it is important to dispel the myth that in fitness the lower intensity aerobic exercises have the effect of keeping an ideal fat burning zone as the anaerobic exercises are more focused on the metabolism on the carbohydrates. It is true that aerobic exercises result to more or fats conversion to calories than carbohydrates; anaerobic workouts have the advantage of putting your body in what is called a post exercise oxygen consumption. At this stage, your body continues to burn calories at an accelerated rate after you are from the gym.

You need to balance both aerobic and anaerobic exercises to be in the right shape and achieve the most out of your time.

Aerobic Methods

Aerobic exercise involves moderate to low intensity physical exertion where the heart rate remains relatively low.

At this point of exercise, the body depends mainly on aerobic metabolism to meet its energy needs, meaning that it requires and is using oxygen. To fully understand this process, it is important to have an idea of how exercise effects various kinds of metabolic pathways in the body.

Generally speaking, during physical exertion muscle glycogen is broken down to glucose which is the main source of energy in the body. Initially, glucose is broken down via an aerobic process called glycolysis and is converted to pyruvate. This energy molecule goes through yet another aerobic pathway which releases energy. If intensity of exercise is maintained at a low level, the body will continue to run on aerobic metabolism for as long as possible and all of the glucose will be converted into energy.

This is the key concept in understanding why aerobic exercise is an efficient way to lose weight and maintain a healthy blood sugar level. As more glucose is converted into energy and glycogen levels begin to be depleted, the liver releases additional glucose into the bloodstream to maintain a healthy blood glucose level and to sustain the energy demands of the body.

Along with this process, fat breakdown also begins. Fat is a high energy molecule and when glucose levels decrease significantly due to aerobic exercise, fat is mobilized from adipose cells and moves into the liver where it is broken down one molecule at a time to generate a high level of energy.

The mobilization of fat molecules is not only important for weight loss, but has also been linked to maintaining proper cholesterol levels and keeping the heart healthy.

At this point, it becomes evident that there is a high level of interplay between the cardiac system and exercise. If level of exercise is maintained at a low to moderate intensity, heart rate remains in a very specific zone where it is higher than resting but not as high as it gets during anaerobic exercise. Because of this, energy demands do not rise above what the bodily supply of glucose is able to maintain, and metabolism never does not go from aerobic to anaerobic.

As a result, glucose is steadily converted to energy for a time, until fat molecules begin to also be utilized. These processes work together to intricately maintain the proper amount nutrition and oxygen available to the body.

A life style that has aerobic exercise as an integral part of its weekly routine, is highly beneficial for losing and maintaining proper weight, as well as for long-term cardiac health.

Regular aerobic exercise not only insures that fat is mobilized and proper fats are present in various tissues, but it also strengthens the heart and respiratory muscles. The heart in particular benefits from this due to something called aerobic conditioning.

In other words, frequent aerobic exercise acclimates the heart muscle into having a higher resting heart rate and stronger heart muscles.

Additionally, aerobic exercise maintains proper blood pressure and improves circulation. The latter benefit is of particular importance as it increases the delivery of oxygen to the muscles and replenishes the ability of cells to maintain proper function.

Overall these benefits add up to very specific health and life benefits. These include reduced risk of cardiovascular disease, reduced risk of insulin resistance and diabetes, reduced risk of bone weakness in older age and reduced risk of obesity. As these diseases are the leading cause of deaths in the Unites States, including 30 - 45 minutes of aerobic exercise every other day as a regular part of the week is very important and may help avoid some serious health issues in the future. Of course, exercise alone will not be sufficient to ward of any of these diseases. A proper and healthy diet must also be maintained at all times.

Together with regular aerobic exercise and good hydration, will keep one healthy and happy for years to come.

In the next chapter we will discuss an exercise regimen so easy; you'll actually want to do this every day!

Chapter 4 – The Get Lean, Fat Burning Routine That Isn't So Mean At All

The hardest thing about developing an exercise routine is usually the "routine" itself, especially for those just starting out. After a long day, taking even a five-minute walk may seem impossible. Take heart, things do get better, just not immediately.

But if you want to lose weight, the first thing you must do is commit.

Commitment is Everything

To build up a routine, it is important to start out easy and stay at a level that you feel comfortable with. Taking on challenges is good, but limit those challenges to only small parts of a workout and make them something that you can handle for more than a day (think of walking for 20 minutes and jogging for ten). You don't want to walk away from a workout feeling so exhausted that you never want to do it again. The body has a way of avoiding pain and the brain is all too ready to agree.

Target Heart Rate – The Key to Fitness

To figure out what exercise level you are at, it is good to start familiarizing yourself with your target heart rate. Don't worry, it's not as complicated as it seems and you only have to do the math once.

Calculating Your Target Heart Rate:

Use 220 if you are a man and 226 if you are a woman. Subtract your age from this number. Here is what the formula would look like for a 50-year-old man.

220-50= 170

In this case, the result of 170 represents the maximum target heart rate. Your target heart rate is somewhere between 50-85 percent of that number. To find the low end of you target heart rate, multiply by 50 percent.

170 x .50= 85 (low)

To find the high end, multiply by 85 percent.

170 x .85= 145 (max)

The key to our recommended program is finding the optimal fat burning zone.

No, this isn't where you exhaust yourself and work yourself to a near heart attack. Your fat burning zone is actually quite lower than an aerobic workout. It's actually listed as between 50 to 60% of your maximum heart-rate

$$170 \times .60 = 102$$

To burn fat at a higher percentage you need to keep your heart-rate between 85 and 102 beats per minute (according to a 50-year old example).

If all of this seems like too much work, you can look to your body for signals instead.

At the low end of your target heart rate, you will just be breaking a sweat. At the high end, you should be sweating profusely. This method is not as accurate, but it will still help you decide when you have reached the "cardio zone."

How do you know if you are burning off that donut?

There is a reason why you need to know your target heart rate. Measuring your heart rate during and after exercise helps to assess how many calories you are actually burning when you work out, and how much fat.

At the peak of your work out, try to count your pulse for ten seconds. You will multiply this number by six to calculate your current heart rate. We know that the above target heart rate is 85. Let's say this pulse beats ten times in ten seconds.

10 x 6= 60 (Heart Rate)

If the goal is to reach 85 and the heart rate is only at 60, then this person isn't working hard enough and it's time to walk a little faster. Why? Because the body doesn't start burning fat until reaching the minimum target of 85 beats per minute (bpm).

Since knowing your heart rate is important and not everyone is good at crunching numbers in their head, you might also consider purchasing a heart rate monitor from the store. This will give you an even better understanding of what your body is doing and how it is improving with more exercise. The more you exercise, the harder your body can push without getting maxed out.

Hurry, Hit the Stop Button

Don't begin a workout routine by trying to hit your maximum heart rate every single time. This kind of activity is strenuous on your body and can be discouraging in the long run. It would be the same thing as deciding that you are going to go on a diet and then not eating for a week. The body cannot handle these types of extremes and it will start to rebel!

Burning Fat vs. Burning Calories

If you jumped out of your chair right now and started to do jumping jacks, your body would immediately start burning up carbs. This is because carbs are a quick source of energy, but your body can only store a limited supply. So what does it burn when it's out of carbs? Fat! This is the reason experts suggest that you should exercise for 20 minutes or more. If you continued to do jumping jacks for the next half hour, your body would start to burn more fat and less carbs in order to maximize its reserve.

Let's look at the case of Bob.

Bob starts jogging in place. This is how his body might break down his energy supply.

First 5 minutes: 70% carbs, 30% fat

After 10 minutes: 50% carbs, 50% fat

After 20 minutes: 40% carbs, 60% fat

Ideally, you want to break that threshold so that you are burning as much fat as possible.

Putting Things Together

To simply summarize what you need to do;

- Commit to a routine
- Start off easy and chose something that you can do 3-5 times a week
- Use your target heart rate to decide how hard you should exercise and for how long
- To maximize fat burning, try to do an activity that you will enjoy for at least 30 minutes.

Exercise doesn't have to be work and you will be surprised at how your body craves it once you are in a routine. Think of something that you enjoy doing every day and how empty your day would seem without it. And there are other benefits to exercising too. When you exercise, your body releases feel good endorphins, making it the perfect way to stave off stress or think through a tricky problem.

Once you have a routine, you will find that you have more energy throughout the day and feel more confident and positive about yourself. You may think of exercise as a chore today, but there are a lot of marathon runners out there who started the exact same way, so don't be afraid to embrace it.

Next, we'll discuss an exercise routine that's so simple; you'll find you can do this for hours without losing your breath!

Chapter 5 – Walking as an AMAZING Secret for Losing Weight

(And why it's actually better than running)

We often turn to exercise as way of burning fat and losing weight because it's cheaper, less complicated, and faster than dieting alone. Any form of exercise ranging from light to rigorous is effective. Therefore understanding what amount of exercise is suitable for you is important to gaining an effective advantage from it. When you intend to burn fat and lose weight, light exercise such as walking is more appropriate than running.

For us to move or perform any task, our bodies require energy. This energy comes from fats and carbohydrates (fuel). Even at rest our bodies consume energy, although at small amounts. When muscle activity increases as we switch from rest to exercise, energy demand also rises. For rest and light exercises our bodies only burn fat to cater for a higher energy demand. As we increase exercise, carbohydrate catabolism (breakdown of complex materials) is initiated. Dependence on carbohydrates as source of energy continues with the rise in intensity of exercise, until it is only the source of energy and the body abandons burning body fats.

If you main goal is to burn fat, walking may be more effective than running.

Low calorie burn-rates

With this low intensity of exercise the rate of burning the calories is low. Therefore, in order to cut down a significant level of fat you will need to exercise for much longer period. When you are starting out on this exercise, you can start with a 20 minute walk and slowly but comfortably increase this time to one hour. As we discussed in the previous chapter, your effective burn-rate of fat is much more efficient when you keep your heart rate in a target fat burning zone rather than attempt to achieve an anaerobic heart rate. At this rate,

79

you exercise your heart much more but fat burning is not as efficiently conducted because the body uses a different fuel source and bypasses burning fat.

You can control the intensity of your light exercise to only target the fat burning zone. This is a zone in which only fat is used for fueling the body. Use a heart rate monitor to determine this zone. This device typically uses a chest strap which communicates information on a special watch. The device calculates the heart rate then utilizes this information to calculate your particular fat burning zone. As you are walking you can monitor the fat burning zone to ensure that the intensity of exercise maintains fat burning zone.

You can attain an optimum intensity by multi-tasking while walking. Here are a few things you can do;

- Engage in conversation with a friend or an acquaintance on the road

- Engaging your brain helps to keep energy demand high because it eats into available energy. This raises your energy demand thus breaking up more fats. Be sure that your heart-rate does not exceed your fat burning zone recommended rate. If your monitor indicates that you have exceeding this zone, then reduce your pace of walking or your participation in the conversation.

- Do other lighter exercises as you walk; you can stretch your hands, or do lighter jogs.

Remember that you are just trying to achieve the optimum fat burning zone but if you find it difficult attaining the optimum zone with additional activities, maintain your walking pace and slowly increase walking time.

Aside from the fact that running will not meet your specific goal of burning fat, walking may still be better than running because of the following additional reasons.

Your body may not be ready physically for running

Recent research found that about 60% of runners had elevated level of cardiac stress serum markers. In particular, Troponin proteins which is a significant part of cardiac muscle; however, high levels of these proteins can cause cardiovascular damage.

Your immune system can be stressed by running

Running, taxes our immune system. Running, especially for long distance, burns fats, but also muscle tissue as well. This places a heavy burden on one's immune system. Running also stresses your spinal discs.

Running particularly in hot weather can cause heat stroke

Excessive running in summer cause multi-organ dysfunction. Walking therefore predisposes you to a risk of heat stroke during this season. With walking you are less likely to have an organ failure in hot weather.

To summarize, walking has many more advantages as an exercise than running. You can achieve substantial amount fat loss and weight loss by walking. Regular walking increases cardiovascular exercise which strengthens your heart and lungs, thus improving overall fitness.

With its low impact, walking carries no risk of injury and yet it offers many opportunities for weight loss as running does. Walking also improves circulation and helps to drain fluid from your lower legs, thus preventing varicose veins.

Walking is the best way to burn fat by keeping your heart rate in your most optimum fat burning zone. Walk with a heart rate monitor to closely

84

track this and aim for one hour to achieve shocking results.

Next we're going to talk about purchasing heart rate monitors and the various types available.

Chapter 6 – Heart Rate Monitors

The secret to optimal fitness is never about the amount of exercise, but rather, it's more about making every session count.

A heart rate monitor (HRM) is a tool used to measure the rate of heart beats per minute. It is used to monitor the cardiovascular highs and lows during competitive or recreational activities.

86

Most models have been designed to keep the heart rate at the optimal levels throughout an exercise. Some HRMs can even alert you when dehydrating or when at a nutritional deficit. Latest models enable data that you can download and analyze through a computer.

Joggers can benefit from heart rate monitors just as athletes do and more can be gained from exercise by aiming to burn more fats. HRMs also help you to maintain your speed as well as target zones, some through audio alerts.

There are 2 main types of heart rate monitors, chest strap models and finger sensors.

Chest Strap Models

By far the most common style, these consist of a chest strap that fastens around the chest and wirelessly transmits continuous heart rate data to a wristwatch-style receiver.

Model features vary widely:

Basic models:

These time your workout and give you continuous, average, high and low heart rate data.

Advanced models:

Many of these submit a coded signal to prevent other HRMs from interfering with your data. They can be partnered with a foot pod that attaches to your shoelaces to track your speed, distance and cadence. Some have GPS receiver capabilities to help you mark/find locations, give elevation and save previous course info.

Pros and Cons

Pros: Chest-strap models offer continuous heart rate information without needing to stop during exercise to measure or view it. Accuracy tends to be better than with finger sensor models, and they offer more options, such as speed and distance monitoring via GPS receivers.

Cons: These are usually more expensive than finger sensor models. Low-end chest-strap models don't prevent crosstalk (interference) with other wireless heart rate monitors. Some chest straps are less comfortable than others.

Finger Sensor Models

These consist only of a wristwatch-style monitor. Simply touch a finger to the unit's touch-pad sensor to activate the heart rate monitor. Finger sensor data is estimated to be 95% accurate.

Pros and Cons

Pros: No chest strap means greater simplicity and comfort. Finger sensor models are more affordable than most chest-strap models.

Cons: You must pause during exercise in order to take a measurement. They tend not to be as accurate as chest-strap models. There is no option for integrated speed and distance monitoring.

Affordable heart rate monitors

Polar FT1 ($45)

It's among the least expensive HRM but performs accurately and is very reliable. Its feature enables you set an intensity zone for your workout; it also has alerts both visual and audible forms and a feature that cuts interference from other devices.

Omron HR-100C ($35)

HOW TO BURN FAT AND LOSE WEIGHT RIDICULOUSLY EASY

This is another HRM that is cheaper but with a few more features, its lack of chronograph deters it from making interval timing but it has a stop watch feature.

Sport Duo 1060 ($85)

This type has a stopwatch, pre-set and custom target zones, additionally it has a speedometer, pedometer and a chest strap too that enables user measure heart rate by placing a finger on the sensor unit.

Models usable with smart phones

Polar H7 Bluetooth Smart Heart Rate Sensor ($60)

This device utilizes smart phones' Bluetooth technology to give the heart rate as a constant display.

Zephyr HxM Bluetooth Wireless Heart Rate Sensor ($75)

This has a combination of a smart fabric, movement sensor, Bluetooth technology and a sensor. This is the first HRM which supports Android and Windows Phone operating Systems. When paired with the phone it gives all the data including speed, distance and GPS location.

60 Beat Bluetooth Heart Rate Monitor ($35)

This one is compatible with iOS operating system and it supports iPhone, iPad mini (4th and 5th generations), iPod touch Nano (7th generation) as well as a variety of Samsung Android enabled phones.

*Note: I personally use a HRM by Beets BLU ($60) which syncs to my Samsung S4. There are apps you can download for free that link to the device which you can use during your workout to stay within your zones.

Now you're probably wondering how long this walking program will take before you see some results. This next chapter will give you some ideas so you can start walking and burning fat right away!

Chapter 7 – How Much Time Will It Take to Get The Weight Off?

When you start a new weight loss program there is never time to waste.

Many people desire to lose weight as early as possible but never relish the thought of waiting for months or days or weeks to significant results.

95

The good news is that some people can see a drastic drop in weight in a very short span of time through this fat-burning program, but keeping in mind that you have to change major lifestyles in order for you to keep your weight balanced.

Experienced weight loss experts recommend following both an exercise approach and calories restriction approach.

In both programs the goal is to lose 1 to 2 lbs. per week, meaning that for you to reach your desired weight it will take approximately one pound drop every week of the weight you want to lose. Although with more disciplined changes it can take a little less time.

The largest weight loss takes place mostly during the first week or the second week of the weight loss program, nevertheless much of that weight is actually water weight. This means that during this first week up to 3lbs of water can be lost in a single exercise like hiking on a humid day.

This means that the first week of weight lose should be devoted to adapting and learning new lifestyle behaviors, eating habits and mastering the daily walking routine. As we discussed previously, walking, unlike the other very many workout programs has been the best way to lose weight and burn fat with the least amount of effort.

What makes walking great is it can be done anywhere!

It doesn't matter what age you are, body chemistry, or current state of fitness; anyone can start this walking program. All it simply takes is to have a pair of a good comfortable sport shoes, a firm resolve, leave the house and start walking.

Brisk walking as an aerobic exercise is very critical in weight loss, in that it can raise your heart beat to even 50 percent of its maximum. This is because it is a whole body activity involving all the muscles of the body (back, legs, shoulders and even buttocks) in a rhythmic fashion at one time making the heart and the entire circulatory system so efficient that it allows more oxygen and nutrients to circulate within the body.

Brisk walking burns up more calories than jogging, you don't even need to walk race like the athletes at the Olympic to feel the effect. You should start off gently and make it regular for three times a week for at least half an hour each session. As you continue you need to reach a point of perspiring and rising in heart beat rate. The easiest way of gauging this is the talk test, being able to pass a word to a friend you working out with but not being at a position to converse as normal.

Preparation

- Set a target but it should be manageable and measurable
- Avoid eating before walking for around an hour; however, if you do, that's still okay
- Drink plenty of water before starting, during and after the exercise
- Start by warm up exercises and stretches to ease the body and make it ready for the

workout

Calorie burn Formula

People are eager to know how much calories they burn in a day comparing with how much they consume to create a calorie deficit that leads to weight loss.

There are several factors to use in measuring this, they include weight, age, heart beat rate, and the rate of workout. Calorie burn formulas can be calculated by wearing the heart rate monitor, which should be tracked to make sure you do not exceed the recommended fat burning zone.

Calorie-burn rate formula for men

Calories burned = [(Age x 0.2017) + (Weight x 0.09036) + (Heart Rate x 0.06309) - 55.0969] x time / 4.8184

Calorie-burn rate formula for women

Calories burned = [(Age x 0.0074) - (Weight x 0.05741) + (Heart Rate x 0.4472) - 20.4022] x Time / 4.184

The bottom line is embrace your own motivation to burn fat and lose weight and use this consistently everyday to make healthy choices in everything you do.

This implies that good health starts in the brain and never in the plate. We have to understand that we never have much control over food as we at times assume. However self-control is a result of a process of decision making. Our will power is our propeller to achieve many things, using it to change our eating habits will work immensely for our benefit. Try to begin it simply by having something simple for breakfast.

Our brains can easily become overwhelmed so try to not develop many habits at once; start with just two or three.

You should stop drinking carbonated beverages and replace them with water and more sugar free vegetable juices.

You should reduce or stop taking alcohol altogether as it makes you store fat easily.

Additionally alcohol is a carbohydrate (sugar) and causes you to store fat.

In all, weight loss is achievable quickly and easily with a few simple strategies.

Keeping a positive attitude and commitment will guide you to the right plan of action on your fat burning strategy. Even positive self-encouraging talk is critical, eating more nutritionally balanced meals, feeling stronger, feeling healthier, and controlling your behaviors will boost self-esteem and encourage you to continue the program, you even can find it easy to resist food temptations only because you have developed a responsible way of living and eating.

A few other tips that are extremely beneficial for fast weight loss while you walk everyday;

- Eat 5-6 small meals per day. Eating more frequently actually increases your metabolism which helps you to lose weight faster. Eat smaller meals more frequently and do not skip breakfast.
- Eat more fiber. Next time you go grocery shopping pay attention to the food label and buy products with higher fiber content. Adding fiber to your diet will help you to lose weight faster by filling you up.
- Drink a glass of water before you eat. Filling up your stomach with water will help suppress your appetite. An extra glass of water will keep you from over eating and help you to lose weight quicker.

- Rather than weigh yourself everyday start measuring around problem areas. A better gauge for fitness is waist size and belly size. It's also faster to see results this way than getting discouraged on the scale.

Chapter 8 – Recommended Intake of Healthy Calories

When developing your strategy to eat right, keep carbs low, and enjoy maximum nutrition, you'll want to select diets that focus on heart healthy options.

Our bodies require a vast amount of energy to perform some of even the simplest tasks. Think of all the processes occurring in your body at any given moment, your heart beating, your digestive tract moving food, your brain firing off impulses in milliseconds…we take all of these things for granted but it's mind blowing to consider for a moment the energy requirements.

Calculating the Body's Energy Stores

So, our first question would be how do we calculate and track energy as a function of daily activity? The basic unit of measurement for this energy expenditure is such a common term, we tend to associate it with something bad that we must avoid, but yet to avoid this unit would bring certain death.

Calories are known to us all as that unit of measurement typically used in conjunction with weight loss (or weight gain for body builders) as a tracking mechanism but what is it really?

According to scientific textbooks, it's actually a unit of heat, specifically what it takes to heat a gram of water one degree Celsius. So why do we care?

Well, calories actually represent how much potential energy that a particular source of fuel (food) will provide the human body.

Energy Production

So let's take a look at the basic building blocks of food, carbohydrates, protein, and fat. A gram of carbohydrates has 4 calories, a gram of protein has 4 calories, and a gram of fat has 9 calories. If you know how many carbohydrates, fats and proteins are in any given food, you can determine how many calories, or essentially, how much energy, that food contains.

So why is it that if calories represent energy, then why would too many cause you to gain weight?

The body is always in a state of burning calories. This burn is actually a metabolic process where enzymes break down carbohydrates into glucose and other sugars, fats into glycerol and fatty acids and the proteins into amino acids. These amino acids are then transported through the bloodstream to the cells, where they are either absorbed for immediate use or sent on to the final stage of metabolism in which they are reacted with oxygen to release their stored energy.

Sounds great as an energy process but we do we gain weight?

Well, too much of a good thing can be a bad thing. Excess amino acids are absorbed through the small intestine's lining and enter the blood stream. From here, some of the amino acids build the body's protein stores; however, the excess amino acids are converted to fats and sugars. Even excess protein turns to fat.

The type of calories consumed is something to watch also. With fat calories, weight gain gets more "bang-for-the-buck" since there are more calories in fat than any other source of fuel. So, by eating fatty foods you're consuming a more dense load of calories than, let's say, plain vegetables, where you would need to eat a roomful to get the same amount of calories. Ok, that last part was an exaggeration but you get the idea.

So are there foods that can actually give you energy?

If you need to boost your energy, you should look at low-glycemic foods because they release energy slowly and are high in complex carbohydrates yet low in excess fats. Iron is also very important because it produces red blood cells that carry blood to exercising muscles (although men should use caution that too much iron may actually be toxic). A first step is to eliminate junk foods that contain simplex carbohydrate foods, like candy bars and sweetened soda, which spike your energy level before it plunges quickly.

Ten foods that you can implement in your eating strategy can help you get back on the road to vitality and provide you the extra energy you need to succeed in life. Perhaps you need the extra energy for school or concentration. Try these simple eating changes and foods to make a difference.

Whole grains are high in fiber which can help slow the breakdown and absorption of sugar as well as complex carbohydrates. They also contain antioxidants similar to those in fruits and vegetables. Additionally, they reduce the risk of cancer, diabetes, and heart disease. Adults should

eat 6 to 11 servings of whole grains per day.
Examples include whole grain breads, pastas, and
rice.

Oatmeal. According to the American Dietetic
Association, oat products are some of the best
sources of soluble fiber. You can combine oatmeal
with raisins, honey, and yogurt for extra flavor and
energy.

Bananas. This fruit is packed with potassium,
which helps your muscles contract. One per day
prevents stiffness that comes from sitting at a desk.

Orange Juice. This drink is ideal for the morning
and is extremely high in vitamin C, which helps
you get the most iron out of other foods.

Salmon. This fish is high in protein, and its high concentration of omega-3 fats and B vitamins can boost your cardiovascular health.

Beans. A small, powerful vegetable packed with protein, fiber, vitamins, and minerals, beans can be used in creative ways. Add them to soups, burritos, pastas, and dip spreads. In 2005 the Department of Agriculture recommended that Americans eat three cups of beans per week.

Dried fruit. These high-energy, low-fat snacks are easy to pack and almost never go bad. Try a medley of apricots, figs, and raisins. However, be aware that some commercially packaged dried fruits contain sulfur dioxide, which has been shown to increase your risk of asthma.

Almonds. Ounce-for-ounce, this is the most nutrient-dense nut. Research has shown that adding two ounces of almonds to your daily diet increases your intake of vitamin-E and magnesium.

Yogurt. Quick, easy, and delicious, yogurt is available in a variety flavors. One cup of low-fat yogurt contains almost 13 grams of protein and 17 grams of carbohydrates-just what you need for great energy.

Antioxidants

We've all heard of the power of antioxidants but what can they really do for us? If we know anything about them, we've all heard that they prevent free radicals from mutating into cells that can eventually turn into cancer but let's take a further look at what they actually are.

Well, from a chemist's point, an antioxidant is a molecule that does exactly what its name suggests, preventing the oxidation of other molecules. Oxidation is a chemical reaction that transfers electrons or hydrogen from a substance to an oxidizing agent. Oxidation reactions can produce free radicals. In turn, these radicals can start chain reactions. When the chain reaction occurs in a cell, it can cause damage or death to the cell.

Recent studies suggest; however, that the benefits of antioxidants are much overstated and can actually be harmful to human longevity. High doses that can be found in supplements can cause some serious side effects such as beta carotene (high concentrations increased the risk of cancer in people who smoke), Vitamin E (risk of prostate cancer), and selenium (skin cancer).

If antioxidants were our last hope, we're screwed, but fortunately this is not the case.

Oxidation Fighting Foods

The food we eat has just the right amount of naturally occurring antioxidants (with a simple whole-food multivitamin just enough to be a safe supplement). Eating foods from the following list and quantities per serving (or dose if you like to still think of it that way) will ensure you are living with the right number of radical-fighters (and inhibit oxidation);

Artichoke (cooked)	1 cup (hearts)	Pinto bean	Half cup
Black bean (dried)	Half cup	Plum	1 whole
Black plum	1 whole	Prune	Half cup
Blackberry	1 cup	Raspberry	1 cup
Blueberry (cultivated)	1 cup	Red Delicious apple	1 whole
Cranberry	1 cup (whole)	Red kidney bean (dried)	Half cup
Gala apple	1 whole	Russet potato (cooked)	1 whole
Granny Smith apple	1 whole		
Pecan	1 ounce	Small Red	Half

Bean (dried)	cup
Strawberry	1 cup
Sweet cherry	1 cup
Wild blueberry	1 cup

Fiber

Fiber is an important consideration in any diet, but little attention is actually given why. Recent studies are proving that diets high in fiber can actually reduce your risk of some cancers, diabetes, digestive disorders, and heart disease. Additionally, most diets suck when it comes right down to it. If you follow a "low carb" diet you will most likely be eating foods that have a difficult time passing through your system such as meat, cheese, and other fatty toxic foods. Sure, these low glycemic foods will help you lose weight fast but it causes havoc on your body as it adjusts to processing the additional protein without the roughage needed to evacuate it from your system.

Fiber also may boost your energy levels but this is an indirect effect of removing toxins from your body that contribute to fatigue and other energy-robbing symptoms.

Proper dose of fiber?

Typically, most men should consume 38 grams of fiber every day and women should consume 25 grams at least. Older men and women, respectively, should eat between 30 and 21 g daily.

High-fiber foods include fruits, vegetables, nuts, seeds and whole grains. You shouldn't be afraid to take a fiber supplement containing psyllium husk or a fiber powder to mix with your morning drink. This will ensure regular, timely toxin removal (bowel movements) and ensure unused food waste is not left in your body.

If you have a high speed juicer, a potent energy/high fiber drink will consist of vegetables pureed into a drinkable concoction. Consider sweetening the drink with berries or another food high in antioxidants (so you can benefit in multiple ways). High-fiber vegetables include carrots, broccoli, cabbage, cucumber, tomatoes and spinach.

Additionally, adding protein powder will create a third powerful way of obtaining a hunger-reducing benefit.

Chapter 9 - Diet Plans for the 21st Century

Today, there many different types of popular plans available which can help you shed further weight but should be used in conjunction with this walking-fitness program.

The following are the most used diet plans currently recommended by physicians;

3 – Hour Diet

The 3-Hour diet requires individuals to eat five times on a daily basis. Individuals are allowed to be taking their favorite foods, including sweets and carbs, so long as they are observing a strict timetable. According to this diet plan, eating small and balanced meals every 3 hours in a day boosts burning of fat in an individual's body. It is argued that eating every 3 hours resets an individual's metabolism, and hence, the individual's body is able to burn fat throughout the day.

The rules around the 3-Hour meal are as follows.

- One is required to eat breakfast within 1 hour of rising.

- One is to eat after every 3 hours after taking breakfast

- One must eat 3 hours prior to going to sleep

An individual should adhere to the recommended portion sizes; each meal of the day should have an average of 400 calories; with dessert as 50 calories, and snacks 100 calories, for a total of approximately 1450 calories a day.

An individual who practices this type of meal plan strictly, should be able to lose up to 10 pounds of weight in the first 2 weeks, and 2 pounds in each of the subsequent weeks. The biggest advantage of this meal plan is that an individual is allowed to continue eating his/her favorite's foods.

http://www.webmd.com/diet/3-hour-diet

The Atkins Diet

The Atkins diet require an individual to objectively cut back on consuming carb, so that the body is able to burn fat and releases ketone by-product to be utilized for production of energy. This kind of meal plan has been researched and found out that it effectively contributes to loss of weight.

The plan for Atkins diet

- An individual should not take more than 20 grams of carbohydrate every day.

- An individual should consume proteins and fat from fish, poultry, red meat, eggs, butter, and also eat vegetable oils.

- An individual should not eat bread, past, grains, starchy vegetable, fruits, or other dairy products other than butter, cream and cheese.

- An individual should not eat seeds, nuts, or legumes like beans, should not take caffeine and alcohol.

With this diet plan an individual is advised that as soon as he/she starts to realize weight loss, he/she can gradually start adding more vegetable, and can include seeds, berries, legumes, nuts and other fruits, whole grains, and wine and low carb alcohol, to his/ her food. Atkins diet is quite an effective way of losing diet.

http://www.healthline.com/health-slideshow/diet-reviews#3

Best Life Diet

This diet requires an individual to go through the following main stages which include;

- Baby steps. An individual should ensure that he/she take in activities to revive his/her metabolism to increase the burning of calories. In this stage an individual should eat breakfast every day rich in fiber and calcium, 100-200 calorie snacks, drink plenty of water and eat 2 hours before he/she goes to bed. Further, the individual should not consume, trans-fat, alcohol, fried food, soda, full-fat milk, white bread and yogurt.

- Get moving step. An individual should maintain his/her weight by each time increasing an activity to at least a level up, while comprehending emotional reasons for hunger. During this stage, an individual should control his/her meal portions depend upon the activity level.

- Your best life step. An individual at this stage is required to cut back on saturated fat, added sugar, sodium, eliminate trans-fat, and add wholesome foods in the diet. At this stage, an individual should shift to nutritious food while keeping portions in check consisting of whole grain, lean proteins, vegetables and fruits. The advantage with this type of diet is that an individual can be cooking and shopping as usual so long as he/she adheres to the guidelines of best life, and additions vitamins and supplements.

http://www.webmd.com/diet/the-best-life-diet

Cabbage Soup Diet

This diet is very effective for losing weight in the first 7 seven days. It is suitable for short-term weight loss. This kind of diet enables an individual to lose weight faster within a week. An individual on cabbage soup diet must follow these things for remarkable weight loss.

Drink a minimum of 4 glasses of water a day

Complement his/ her diet with quality day-to-day multivitamins.

Eat plenty of cabbage soup

Add a variety of spices to the soup to make it taste better.

An individual's diet on this plan must consume cabbage soup for a week so that he/she loses about 10 pounds of weight in a week. For example, the individual can adhere to the following procedure

- Day 1. Consume cabbage soup and plenty of fruits except bananas to his/ her satisfaction

- Day 2. Consume cabbage soup and any types of vegetables, either cooked or raw.

- Day 3. Consume cabbage soup and plenty of fruits and vegetables to his/her satisfaction

- Day 4. Consume cabbage soup and 8 bananas, and skimmed milk to his/ her satisfaction

- Day 5. Consume cabbage soup and up to 20 ounces of beef, fish, and/or skinless chicken.

- Day 6. Consume cabbage soup and beef, fish and/or skinless chicken to his/her satisfaction.

- Day 7. Consume cabbage soup and brown rice, unsweetened fruit juice and vegetables without potatoes.

The advantage of this diet plan is that you can lose weight fast and quick; however, you must include exercise as part of your daily routine.

http://www.healthline.com/health/cabbage-soup-diet

Paleo Diet

This diet plan requires an individual to be taking large quantities of proteins and fiber to cut weight. In this diet an individual can eat plenty of fresh lean meat, fruits, fish, healthier fat and vegetables. However, an individual is restricted not to eat any processed food and also, avoid refined sugar food, dairy, salt, potatoes and refined vegetable oils. An individual on this diet will need to stock up only the accepted food, and not to shop for any type of processed food. This diet primarily emphasizes eating of fish and lean meat and low salt food.

http://www.webmd.com/diet/paleo-diet

Fat Flush Diet

This diet plan requires an individual to follow through three phases, which are;

Phase 1. An individual only takes 8 glasses of cranberry juice and water mixture every day to reduce retention of water. In addition, an individual should be taking 1100-1200 calories a day, and avoiding dairy products and wheat.

Phase 2. An individual is required to slightly add small amounts of carbohydrate in the diet.

Phase 3. An individual requires practice a diet ratio of 30% protein, 40% carbohydrate and 30% fat.

Furthermore, fat flush diet encourages an individual to engage oneself in doing body exercises to facilitate loss of weight.

http://www.diet.com/g/fat-flush-diet

Chapter 10 – Stay (Hydrated) My Friends!

When you go to the gym or head out for a run, it's likely that you have a bottle of water with you or at least know where the water fountain is. Whether you are properly hydrated or not does not depend on whether you have water for your workout. If you go to the gym and find yourself getting seriously thirsty, you are not properly hydrated, and it doesn't matter how much water is in your bottle (or in the fountain). Hydration is a process that you have to continue all day long, and keeping your water levels appropriate will boost your health in a number of ways.

Why is hydration so important?

If you weigh 155 pounds, your body has approximately 11 gallons of water in it if you are properly hydrated. Those 11 gallons weigh in at about 92 pounds, meaning that you are about 60 percent water. If you start to dehydrate, you'll notice the effects fairly quickly.

Maintaining supple skin

When you are dehydrated, your skin loses some of its elasticity. This is a different phenomenon from dry skin, which is the sum result of hot water, soap

137

and dry air in the atmosphere. However, if you are properly hydrated, you will feel your skin is a bit softer and more pliable to the touch.

Promoting cardiovascular health

When you go into dehydration mode, your blood volume decreases. This means that your heart has less blood to work with to distribute the oxygen that your body needs. Your heart has to do more work to get the same amount of oxygen out, making the activities that you do every day, such as going upstairs, picking up your children, or washing the car, more strenuous. Over time, the toll on your heart can be significant.

Keeping you from getting dry mouth

If you drink enough water, your lips and throat will stay moist, and your mouth won't get that dry sensation. If your mouth dries up, you can suffer from awful breath and a bad taste in your mouth. In some cases, you can develop cavities if your mouth stays too dry.

Helping you keep your cool

When your body gets too hot, it releases heat through the expansion of blood vessels near the surface of the skin (this is the reason for that redness in your face when you are working out). The end result is a higher level of blood flow, sending heat to the air. When you don't have enough water in your system, the temperature around you has to be higher for your blood vessels to automatically widen, so it's harder for you to stay cool.

Cleansing toxins out of your body

Water is the substance that kidneys use to filter the waste substances from your blood stream and send them into your urine. A lack of hydration can make this process tougher, and it also can elevate your risk of kidney stones and urinary tract infections. If your dehydration becomes serious enough, your kidneys run the risk of shutting down altogether, and the toxins will swiftly build up, leading to an extremely serious condition.

Lubricating joints and muscles

When your hydration is sufficient, the cells that surround your muscles have less waste lodged in them, because the water inside those cells has brought enough nutrients and gotten rid of the toxins. The end result is improved performance. A similar benefit helps your joints move more easily when your hydration levels are good.

Giving you an energy boost

A lot of times, people feel a major drop in energy about an hour after lunch. They go from feeling energetic to craving a nap in a matter of minutes. While many people turn to snacks or candy to give them an energy boost, dehydration can also be the culprit. Water helps your blood get your cells the oxygen they need, as well as the essential nutrients. Keeping your water levels up helps you

141

feel a more even level of energy throughout the day.

One of the best ways to keep hydrated all day long is to keep a water bottle with you. If your workplace offers access to bottled water, keep refilling your own bottle throughout the day, so that hydration becomes a habit, not a necessity to satisfy your thirst.

Conclusion

I hope you found this eBook useful for starting your walking program. Walking as a way of fitness is something people consider too small of an activity to gain any advantage in losing weight and burning fat; however, the secret is in the fat burning zone and closely monitoring your heart rate. Do not let your heart-rate go outside the zone and if this happens, don't be afraid to slow down.

I was a runner jogging an average of 5 miles per day but when I discovered the secret of the fat burning zone, I decided to pursue this as a routine because of the substantial benefit of burning fat calories first.

At first I was disappointed because I felt like I wasn't getting anything out of it; but after walking for an hour "in the zone" I noticed an immediate difference. I came home STARVING, and I mean ravenously starving. This is how I knew it worked. The best thing to do if you encounter this craving is to have a protein shake immediately to suppress your appetite until you can rationally prepare a healthier but smaller meal later on in the evening.

One thing to always remember is to NEVER lose hope and give up. Every time you walk or make a healthier choice to take the stairs instead of the elevator, you are always doing something to better your life. The secret to weight loss and looking good is to make small changes every day, no matter how hard it may seem.

Always set goals! I strive to do this even though there will be hiccups in your schedule and you may have to delay your routine for a day due to some emergency. These things happen but it doesn't mean you should quit.

Give yourself a reward when you've managed to hit a goal. Whether it's hitting a certain weight loss goal or even an inch from your waist, it's okay to celebrate! Milestones are a great thing and should be applauded, even if it's only you doing the applauding.

No matter how much time you can allocate to your walking routine you should do it. Never tell yourself that only 10 minutes isn't worth it or giving up easily. Always be doing something to keep moving yourself to a new you!

Finally, a great way of keeping a routine is to include family, friends, and significant others in your new walking program. In reaching the fat burning zone, you can still maintain a conversational pace (which means you should not be out of breath in this zone). This is an incredible way to catch up with a friend, play trivia games, or just relax in someone else's company.

Remember, starting small is the key and keeping your heart-rate in the right zone for over 20 minutes is the secret to the success of this ridiculously easy walking program.

Gerry Marrs

About the Author

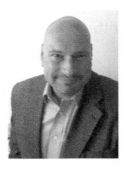

Gerry Marrs is a research analyst who enjoys helping people and giving back to his community. He started a homeless meals program in his neighborhood which is now on complete auto-pilot, serving free meals to over 400 local homeless vets and those who struggle with addictions each month. He enjoys writing in his spare time on a variety of topics and hopes to build a successful portfolio of "how to" products designed to help people struggling with a variety of issues.

He is currently working on a Ph.D. in Business Administration and while not immersed in dissertation writing, is raising two successful kids and loves Disney World. He currently lives on the Gulf Coast in Florida along the world's most beautiful beaches.

Made in United States
North Haven, CT
14 June 2023

37749384R00085